My Garden
of Intimacies

TARA GREEN

BALBOA.PRESS
A DIVISION OF HAY HOUSE

Balboa Press books may be ordered through booksellers or by contacting:

Balboa Press
A Division of Hay House
1663 Liberty Drive
Bloomington, IN 47403
www.balboapress.com.au
AU TFN: 1 800 844 925 (Toll Free inside Australia)
AU Local: 0283 107 086 (+61 2 8310 7086 from outside Australia)

Print information available on the last page.

ISBN: 978-1-9822-9122-8 (sc)
ISBN: 978-1-9822-9123-5 (e)

Balboa Press rev. date: 07/29/2021

Dedicated to my children who expected nothing less than for me to fly high, take risks and live life to the absolute fullest...

CHAPTER ONE

I've already had one whole life of love, losses and many unfulfilled and misunderstood moments of desire. So, when I was free of the first life I began to ask myself, what do I want to do at 62 onward and do differently in this second time around.

I began to hear stories from women about my age and even younger who gathered around to tell me I was entering a defining age where I could expect to lose energy, lose vitality, lose my looks, my body, my ambition, my sexual drive and my confidence.

I listened but the information I was being fed didn't seem to match the way I felt at 62 and still doesn't match at 73.

I was told now is the time to start wearing beige, be a little less visible...kick off those stilettos and get comfortable in some flat shoes. Know that going to bed early and meeting the girls for coffee once a week is what you dream about and life will start revolving around medications and doctors appointments.

REALLY?

Maybe I'm doing something wrong because life has and continues to revolve around hot steamy sex with incredibly long and satisfying orgasms, stiletto heels, deep heart felt connections and intimacies. Some relationships are long and ongoing, some short, some heart expanding and opening and some heart breaking but my heart has deep memory and feelings and it's bursting with the most fantastic stories and I still have time to fit in a coffee here and there!

I recognised that if the model presented to me didn't fit I would have to create a new model or a new paradigm for moving forward. I asked myself, what do I need? What do I want? Are there any beliefs that I want to take forward in this new creation? Is it possible to create a "new belief system," embracing all possibilities and potentialities my belief in quantum physics and manifesting leads me to believe it is possible.

So I'm now looking at myself and recognising the incredible wealth of wisdom, knowledge and fearlessness I have. I feel like a full blown Goddess who has finally come into her own. I know I am enough...I know I am complete, and I know I have no insecurities or pain that I can't overcome. And I have a T - shirt that says FEARLESS .....and I wear it!

I have researched a new way to live through creating a "new way", a new path or another model. Having no known role models to follow I began to create something for myself and perhaps other women who might want to go forward dipping their toes into the waters of deeper more fearless connections and intimacies. I've read and studied:

- chakra opening
- tantric pathways
- sensuality
- sexuality
- creative processes
- intimacy
- ritual and ceremony
- polyamory
- open relationships

- monogamy
- Gods and Goddesses
- energy
- compassion…

I've taken journeys
inward…outward…upward…downward…around and through…
I would say I have looked for and found my "animal soul", as A.H. Almass states:

> "When we finally confront this powerful aspect of the soul we find a dimension of our self that is very energetic but has a minimum of structure." Almass also says, our normal inner experience of ourselves is in the shape of the body and is actually the result of the development of ego structures that structure the soul through imprinting her with self image whose primary component is an image of body. So, when we fully experience the animal dimension or (total surrendering) of our soul we are going beyond our normal structure or more accurately revealing a part of ourselves that has never been structured.

So, if I can appreciate and not fear the unstructured "animal soul" and understand that this is exactly what we are tapping into in our most powerful intimacies fearlessly releasing all structure, fear, constraints and need for commitment and structure then I am in the best place possible for the best intimacies of a life-time. With this acknowledging that we are animals and like animals we want variety, multiple relationships offer me multiple opportunities to satisfy many parts of myself.

So, I'm thinking it's virtually an impossibility that one person could offer me or I could offer them everything. It is a huge responsibility for any one person to fulfil all my needs or me theirs. One person may be compatible for:

- Living together and making a home
- Another to travel and take risks with
- Another to dream with
- And another to dance and create with

In choosing to be monogamous I would be telling one person (only one person) that I would love only them, I would deny myself the love of all others.

We as humans have a huge capacity to love and a huge capability to love many and for many different reasons. Why do we choose to deny ourselves of extended multiple intimate relationships. Again, we mostly choose to put enormous pressure on ourselves and our partners to provide everything. We humans generally have a large circle of loving friends, we don't tell our friends sorry I already have one friend to love I can't have other friends.

Having had a very long monogamous marriage of 30 something years I vowed never to go into another monogamous relationship I told myself it was unnecessary.

At 62 I was free from marriage.

At 62 I also met Lane a single never married childless man half my age. He was exciting, fun, loving and adventurous, very sexy and very intimate with me. I thought what a great affair to have coming out of a complicated long marriage. I never dreamed it would become more than an affair, but it did. My relationship lasted a little more than 5 years. It was exhilarating to take the ride with a younger attractive man who thought I was pretty special. Lane thought I was amazing and said so and treated me so. But, after about 2 years the affair turned into daily

4

life together and daily routine. While having many friends we had no other lovers! We had become monogamous while I wasn't even looking and weren't satisfying one another's needs.

It was at that time in the later part of our time together that I began to question the "fairytale".

You know the "fairytale" that generation after generation keep falling for.

The repeatable pattern of finding our "ONE SOULMATE" who can offer us everything and we them. In sickness and health, for richer for poorer, till death do us part! You know the drill!

I now realised if I completely rejected this model I would have to create a new model and a new belief system. Creating a new definable belief system and way of navigating it became really important, interesting and exciting for me.

I was beginning to really sharpen my listening skills with all humans men and women. I began to develop heart meditations on a daily basis. Trying to sync my heart to my brain to harmonise and bring coherence. I began testing out how it feels to make most decisions from my "heart" not my "head" the more I practiced the better I got at listening.... I listened to the words, the expressions and the body language. The more I listened, the more I heard the needs of people. I listened with no judgment and I recognised that a new paradigm for relationships was emerging for me. An intimacy of love, trust, truth, transparency and multiple relationships.

I began wanting to go into multiple relationships letting the person know I was there to give unconditionally to them and that I would ask for nothing. Also, if there was chemistry enough to have a second date I let them know I would be having multiple relationships. I asked how they felt about it. I issued invitation to a new way of thinking and a new way of being in a relationship and most importantly new fresh dialoguing.

Lots of important conversations have developed over the last eleven years. It has become abundantly clear to me that many humans are lonely and fearful, fearful that we will lose more than we will gain in entering a relationship. Yet we are lonely so, given the choice yes, we would rather multiple relationships based on a currency of truth and transparency not one based on "what the other"has to offer us. But, like sheep to slaughter we follow an outmoded paradigm that offers only a 50% success rate and a 97% chance that you and your partner/ soulmate will cheat on each other. And all to have someone to call your own. I've decided to go into a relationship asking for nothing other than the currencies that are important and truly valued.

- Immediacy
- Intimacy
- Time
- Truth
- Transparency and being in the absolute present moment!
- Never dragging or dipping into the past which is only "interpretation" or projecting into the future which is "illusion".

What if, just what if we humans were able to walk away from our time together and feel like it was enough, we were enough, the experience was enough. What if we didn't ask each other, the morning after question,"where is this going?"

Perfect timing to meet David, he is a practicing poly and we meet in another country where we both live on and off and have over the past 4 years. David was forty eight when we met. I would call David devoted to being single and having variety in his life. He is sensitive to sound, light and emotional conflict. He is impatient and quick to anger yet he gets his feelings hurt very easily. We talk about everything…he makes no apologises about saying his favourite topics are sex, drugs and rock and roll! He at the same time is romantic and one touch of his hand on my thigh makes me feel loved and protected.

Riding on the back of his motor cycle is exhilarating, I like to arch my back and press up against him, he grabs my thigh and then pulls over on the side of the road, its pitch dark and we are riding through a road cut in the jungle. David says take your helmet off and let the wind blow through your hair and touch your face, now smell the jungle! We pull back out onto the road with some eccentric heavy metal music blasting in the night jungle. He is my partner to take risks with.

He makes no apologies for having multiple relationships and he is very practiced and good at it. We still have an amazing ongoing relationship which is 4 years old, its still open, honest, exciting and totally unpredictable. David loves all types of women but he doesn't like complication or drama.

When he wakes up with a women in the morning and she asks "where is this going", his answer is always the same. It's going right here where we are in the moment. But if you can enjoy this moment and stay in the moment there are likely to be many moments and intimacies maybe even four years worth or a lifetimes worth.

At the time of writing this we are still connecting on many different levels in different countries. We make sure we are accessible to each other to share our joys and our stories. David is the easiest man to say I love our friendship and I miss you without complication or ever entering into the future.

A man named Evan enters my life next, Evan was thirty nine when we met. From the beginning we liked to tell each other our stories. We have both been absolutely transparent starting from the platform of truth and respect. When it became apparent that we were both moving

toward an intimacy with each other I said to him…I'm polyamorous…
I have other lovers. I ask him how he felt about that. He remarked "I
haven't personally experienced that before but I trust you, so I'm going
to go with it."

I planned a ceremony for our first time together. Flowers, incense,
candles, singing bowls, chakra openings, chanting and breathing
techniques but, first I ask him if he had any boundaries and if so what
were they? I had already felt that Evan was a viable lover bringing
him into the fold would only upgrade my current situation with an
abundance of currencies that really mattered to me …growth, higher
consciousness, awareness and an evolution of the soul.

He also offered me the freedom of loving unconditionally. Evan was
and still is a beautiful dreamer and co-creator of this Universe. Someday
he would like to partner full -time with someone and have a child, we
both feel everything we do in the here and now together supports this
happening in his future. Some time into this beautiful relationship Evan
communicated to me that he wasn't keeping up with me and said, he
needed to upgrade his circuitry. Evan made me aware of how powerful
we were together and how this energy needed correct intention and
direction. I thought we were landing our hours of intimacies perfectly
but I didn't notice he wasn't, he was exhausted and unable to focus on
his work the next day. I was pretty stunned that I hadn't felt this or
sensed this. It wasn't long before he injured himself which took a year of
recovery and reflection for both of us. I began to realise how important
all the conversations we had over that year were. I needed to not stare,
but look, not look but truly see what this wonderful human was going
through. It was important to:

- make no assumptions
- ask for nothing

- give everything
- and above all listen and be patient…

At one point I remember saying, we don't need to keep being lovers we started as friends, let's go back to being friends. He very clearly said, that's not what I'm asking for. I'm asking for time to work on myself to be able to land our intimacies I need to be more grounded and more earthed. We are still navigating this terrain and unpacking our time together and we have decided in the near future our intimacies need to be ceremonial, ritualistic and contain definite intention toward spiritual development. What an opportunity for me to grow and what a privilege and honour to listen to how I can better serve someone I care so deeply about.

I've travelled back to the other country that I live part time. In a few weeks David will be back in town and we are looking forward to seeing each other. While sitting at a cafe one afternoon I meet Barry we literally saw each other from across the room as corny as that sounds and couldn't take our eyes off one another. Instant chemistry and instant attraction. We spent the next five hours talking and touching each other much to the amusement of the waiters around us. When it was time to go we both wanted more so we decided to meet again that evening after my rehearsal.

I set up my villa and bedroom with flowers, candles and incense. This has become an important ritual for me along wth tantric kundalini music. We were both like children so excited to see one another. I took Barry by the hand and walked him downstairs to my bedroom unbuttoned his shirt pulled my dress over my head and dropped it to the floor. We kissed each other so passionately and we had the most magical night together neither of us wanted it to end…. I was flying out in the morning to do something in another city and he was continuing his travels… moments of magic with no beginning and no end. That was several years ago. Barry and I still write poetry and love letters to each other and send nourishing photo's. If, we ever have the opportunity to meet again we will and it will be pure sensual magic and childish romantic play. Just two days ago we expressed to each other: wouldn't it be fantastic to be in the same place at the same time again, one of those little Hawaiian islands would suit both of us just fine.

Back in my hometown eight weeks later I meet Blake for a first date…after a few really fun hours together talking and laughing I left for an appointment. We exchanged numbers and an hour later I received this message. "Best first date ever," and I've had a lot of first dates he said, please meet me tonight and we can go to a show. We saw that show and went to dinner, Blake was charismatic and funny and there was definitely chemistry. He asked me to stay the night with him. I had never slept with anyone on a first date so, I decided as part of my education I would see what that felt like. It was great! I had no preconceived notions nor did I suffer from any guilt or social stigma that said you shouldn't be doing this. Remember I'm from a generation that wouldn't have thought of doing such a thing. It was a wild and memorable night together. His parting words were, "I'm an emotional procrastinator!" Haha!…he disappeared for a year to his home country and then reappeared one year later for another fun night together. He is my once a year guy and it's about time for him to reappear again but he is not a viable human to have a deep and meaningful ongoing poly relationship with and I understand that. But all relationships no matter how long or short are teachers especially if we can lead from the heart and risk everything.

In the "Forty rules of love", Elif Shafak says, "Intellect and love are made of different materials… Intellect ties people in knots and risks nothing, but love dissolves all tangles and risks everything." Blake definitely lives in his head not his heart. Then she writes this beautiful passage, "The path to truth is a labour of the heart not the head." "Make your heart your primary guide not your mind." "Meet, challenge and ultimately prevail over your Nafs with your heart."

Perfect spiritual love food for me to digest before meeting Dane a big man with a big bald head which I have grown to find very sexy. Appearance wise a bit raw but with a very soft and calm voice. Our first date was drinking chai together in a coffee lounge. We share a love of chai! I felt relaxed and comfortable as did he on our first date but I wasn't convinced there would be a second date until we kissed on the sidewalk outside. Dane was an unbelievably good kisser and heaps of sparks and sparkles flew. We meet again for a second date at my place, where I make home made chai and set a fire. We had an incredibly beautiful intimacy which was so stimulating it ungrounded me…for the first time I understood what Evan had been feeling…I was a bit overwhelmed and when he called the next day I told him I was ungrounded in fact I was trying to figure out if this relationship was something I could handle. I knew it could teach me but I wasn't sure if I was ready for the teachings as I knew it would be a new deeper more intimate level of surrendering. If I was honest with myself I would have to admit it had already began to teach me.

So I said yes, and dived in. Dane has been my biggest emotional challenge so far. He is an amazing lover.. kind, giving, loving and walks on the wild side. Every time we are together he gives selflessly to me, like no one has ever done before. Its always all about me and my needs. He has become my totally fulfilling man physically but emotionally I was challenged and in the process of recognising this I realise he is my absolute learning ground for true surrendering. He is my man of the moment always and only. He disappears often but comes back always. I've learned to ask no questions and we don't need to talk, could this actually be the ultimate surrendering, trust and transparency? All I need to know is he opens my heart but also is capable of breaking my heart. I continue to engage because I'm learning to go "deeper down the rabbit hole of mysteriousness".

Tristan Taormino, writes about the "fairytale" in "Opening Up", he says, "it's no wonder people are so dissatisfied monogamy sets most people up to fail." "The rules of traditional monogamy are clear you've vowed to be emotionally and sexually exclusive with one person forever." But it's the unspoken rules that will trip us up. "We've collectively been sold a fairytale of finding that one person with whom you'll live happily ever after."

The expectations are endless: your one and only is your soulmate, the person with whom you are 100% sexually and emotionally compatible your "other half" with whom you share the same values about everything. He or she will fulfil all your needs:

- physically
- emotionally
- psychologically
- affectionately
- financially
- romantically
- sexually
- and spiritually.

If you are truly in love, you will never have any desire for anything from anyone else!

Having had a thirty something year complicated long marriage I recognised how unrealistic and unattainable this was. Not to mention the expectation that we would grow together at the same rate and in the same direction. Since there aren't many manuals or scripts for multiple or open relationships if we are going to engage in them we have to create our own version which will ultimately be different for everyone depending on our own level of "comfort" and "creativity". I have days of feeling more comfortable and more creative and I have days of feeling the chaos of juggling multiple relationships but basically I know that nothing stays the same and this polyamory can morph and change to meet my growing needs and the needs of my partners.

Christopher age twenty-nine unexpectedly enters stage right!

Ridiculous the age difference right? Thats what I said, but when I presented my case of age differential to Christopher and said why couldn't you be twenty years older he remarked why can't you just be in the moment! Well…you've got me I said…besides we both share a love of shallot pancakes!

Our first date I ask him five questions and he asked me five questions a fun game I like to play. His first question to me was, what is your favourite colour? I said, navy blue. He started kissing me passionately, I pulled away for a moment and said with a giggle you don't know much about me to which he said, I know your favourite colour is navy blue from that point on we have continued to see each other whenever one of us reaches out and we enjoy fantastic intimacies and conversations without any complications.

I briefly went out with Nathan while holidaying in another country, we still write to each other occasionally and it's a short but flowing conversation of "hows my sexy woman", "how's my sexy man", that's it, pleasant memories of a short 3 week holiday. I'm always happy to receive these short sweet messages which contain no more decoding than the obvious.

At the moment I'm having conversations with two interesting men Erik and Kevin. We will see where this journey goes, both are in relationships with women whom they are married to but all concerned have agreed to "open relationships", venturing into this territory is new for me and what I've learned already is that "open relationships", doesn't always mean it comes without insecurities, judgements and jealousy, these are still things that need to be worked on. Having gone on a first date and really connecting deeply with someone doesn't mean the wife although having agreed changes her mind out of jealously at this deep connection. As she creates new rules for her insecurity I'm ask to wait until they sort out their stuff. I can easily do that or step away completely because what this has done is offer all of us an opportunity to see where our lines of comfort and chaos lie, where the fluctuations of our minds over our hearts are dictating our choices our futures and our happiness. All of this said, this journey still holds windows of opportunity and worlds of potentiality.

For me intimacy is a sacred act of spiritual loving and giving where I treat you like the "divine being" that you are and you treat me like the "Shekinah," the Indwelling presence, that I am…

Elif Shafak offers her last and "fortieth rule of love", "A life without love is of no account. Don't ask yourself what kind of love you should seek, spiritual or material, divine or mundane Eastern or Western… Divisions only lead to more divisions. Love has no labels, no definitions. It is what it is, pure and simple."

"Love is the water of life.

And a lover is a soul of fire!

The universe turns differently when fire loves water."

And this is just the beginning…

CHAPTER TWO

To Love a Woman...

Love doesn't need to make sense, it is what it is. Love is neither this nor that and it doesn't wear labels well. But, in saying that I can't deny that loving another woman is much, much different than loving a man.

More and more I find it's not the gender I'm falling in love with but rather the human who just happens to wear a particular gender suit. I have fundamentally believed this for quite some time but haven't had many opportunities until recently to live with this and feel this to be my truth.

I've been fortunate enough and very surprisingly and unexpectedly happy enough to fall in love with another woman.

Simply by following my heart and saying yes to something that was unknown, unexpected and even a bit uncomfortable, I was able to experience what I'm feeling and living now.

Let me go back to 1993, to when my daughter and I decided to take a girls trip to an exotic little fishing town in the north of Australia. I told her she could orchestrate every aspect of our holiday trip. This is what my daughter and I refer to as a "queens holiday" meaning, no boys aloud, she gets to choose where we stay, what we eat, when we eat, and where we eat! She was also in charge of what the landscape of each day would look like. Basically she was in control of all our experiences. She got to choose what movies we watched, what time we went to bed and what time we woke up. Best holiday ever…for both of us.

One day while browsing the markets my daughter stopped in front of a book stall, my eyes looked directly into a book called "The Celestine Prophecy", by James Redfield. Intriguing! I was astounded by what I was reading as it seemed to legitimise the way I was already living my life. One of the profound things about this book was it's encouragement to say "yes" to almost everything. This I well and truly had down pat, imagine the very thing I had been so deeply criticised for in my marriage was the very thing I was now being encouraged to do more of. Many teachers believe a student finds them when she is ready and a student believes the teacher will appear at the perfect time! This book appeared at the correct time, the universe through my daughter pointed me in the absolute right direction. "The Celestine Prophecy," was saying if you say YES you open up all possibilities and potentialities. If you say NO, you eliminate all potentialities and possibilities.

This certainly gave me the juice I needed to keep trusting my instincts and my "YES" choices rather than cutting everything off before it began. YES, was bound to always lead me somewhere interesting… NO, was a dead end.

Not only that, "The Celestine Prophecy", offered 9 insights that I connected with deeply.

- Meaningful coincidences
- The world has a "spiritual design"
- Subtle energy
- Competition for energy
- Energy abundance
- Getting clear
- Using intuition

- Relating to others
- Conscious evolution

I was already years into Mindfulness, Yoga and Energy training so I really resonated with what I was reading. I continued daily life even more actively employing this belief. YES, took me all over the world teaching many different peoples from many different countries. From Australia to Miami to Atlanta to Utah to Colorado to Croatia to Barcelona to Bali to Budapest and India and my most favourite of all cities Istanbul! The colours textures and smells intoxicated me I felt so alive and so nourished by these YES experiences. So, eleven years ago when I became single I took this YES approach to life into a newly emerging personal/ intimate life. It became the foundation to my newly designed way of seeing relationships. Of course in 1993, I had no idea it would lead me to this lifestyle and belief system that I hold to be truth for me now.

So, in the middle of happily navigating a heterosexual polyamorous (slightly pre covid) life I get a text from a woman I really only know on a professional level. The text says, "I want to study with you, would you consider letting me stay with you for ten days and immerse myself in your yoga and the country life style?" My first thought was Hummmm I have just gotten everything organised in my home and in my life so I can go to the other country I live part time. I thought I was clever organising this so I could essentially run away at the drop of a hat! My second reaction and my instincts told me if I said, NO I would be playing it safe and never know the possibilities it might bring. So, I followed my heart and said YES, after all it was only ten days.

Ten days would eventually change everything though but, I didn't know that or couldn't possibly know that at the time. After all isn't this where real growth comes from? The ability to sit with this discomfort and watch yourself squirm and grow.

So, like the lobster who grows so uncomfortable in his ill fitting shell that he sheds it and starts to grow a brand new one I let go and start a new beginning squirming and growing, growing and squirming happily.

As Maze gets settled into her new home for a ten day retreat we decide to structure each day with practices. First up, morning yoga practice 7:30-9:00am followed by a ritualistic walk to find almond milk cappuccino's and do more talking about life and the universe than I could ever imagine a 30 year old would be interested in. After all this is the time of chaos for most 30 year olds. Time for lots of imbalanced chaos and being the centre of your universe. Looking outward not inward. But not Maze she seemed to be looking inward and was interested in answering the 3 little questions that my Guru said were most important in life….. Who am I? What am I doing? Where am I going? We did heart harmonisation and coherence meditations together, we danced, we talked, we laughed a lot, we talked more, cooked dinner, sang and chanted and I started to care a lot! Not just hold compassion and love as I try to do for every sentient being but rather care deeply.

As Australia and the world began to brace themselves for the full brunt of this new and different time that we were approaching and limitations began to be set upon us we looked at it as an incredible time for self loving and self examining. Actually this time became a rare opportunity with fertile ground for growing individually and together. A ten day retreat for Maze had now turned into a full time living arrangement.

With an unpredictable future we decided to help each other and support each other. It was actually exciting as neither of us had ever in our lives had this much time to look inward and move upward and outward with developing ideas and new workshops and ways of teaching, learning and creating. Gaia and Mind Valley lectures were on the daily menu. We shared stories, lots of stories, stories of our pasts both nuclear relationships and partnered relationships. We did some projecting into the near future but mostly we stayed in the moment.

Imagine someone also interested in reading Ram Das, "Be Here Now", how random. As I began to talk about him being my first spiritual influencer and the book that took me through University life in the 70's and not only shaped it but kept me sane, Maze was fascinated and ordered the book and burned through it, all the while decoding all the wonderment of his words and philosophy.

We shared ideas for "workshops with a difference," where opening the heart and letting the spirit soar were as important as weaving stories and deconstructing techniques. Flow and sequentiality were as important as taking risks and growing. Balancing the continuum of the sacred and the mundane and seeing how we could breathe life into new ways of moving and learning that opened the chakras and nourished the heart. Feeding people vegan food prepared with love and socialising and sharing stories began to build towers of healing.

We shared with our small community pretty much on a daily basis as the new way of living without touching began to take hold. We put on unicorn headbands, bunny ears and dressed up to walk into the centre of our little town waving at passerby's to make contact, smiling and a bit of dancing in the streets and on the sidewalks. We did elicit smiles and conversation and generally made people laugh. Although, short on money we were long on smiles and we vowed to each other to get in our daily walk for a takeaway cappuccino. Each day we made people laugh, we started new classes and new sharing's in yoga and dance, we made new friends of all ages.

Our conversations began to travel through new territories and terrains including intimacies, connections and relationships. We talked about unconditional loving, giving and receiving. We both agreed we were in a place where we wanted to say YES to most everything and NO to few things as this is where the growth and many surprises lie. Maze was in a great listening place about the concept of saying YES. When I mentioned the "Celestine Prophecy", she looked shocked and said I haven't read it but I just ordered it for a friend of mine! These meaningful coincidences continued to happen to us over and over.

Our relationship couldn't be defined nor explained nor did it need to be.

One day while sitting out in the back yard in our favourite bright aqua plastic chairs under an umbrella talking and reading, reading and talking Maze said have you ever been with a woman? I had to admit I had once. I had not censored any conversation we have had since she moved in so I couldn't very well start now. She asked what it was like and as I drew from my memory as it had been many years, I remembered it was pretty wonderful, nothing was missing! It was whole and complete and we laughed about if men really understood this it would change the whole dating dynamic. She admitted she was curious and wanted to have this experience for herself one day. I thought about it for weeks and we had a few more conversations leaning in toward the sensations and feelings of being with another woman and what it would feel like.

To be honest I'm not sure where I got the guts from but one day we were both in the kitchen pre morning walk post yoga/meditation practice and I grabbed her and kissed her, she kissed back but then said, I didn't see that coming and I need time to think about it. I said, let's do our walk to town and talk about it. We did walk and talk and what I remember most was both of us were just trying to serve each other with no pressure no right, no wrong. I couldn't help but think if this happened between a man and a women there might have been hurt feelings, misunderstandings and feelings of rejection. Messy.

But there was no messiness here it was just a sense of let us look at our needs and see if this serves us and if not we let it go, there will be someone else who in the future will offer you this experience. About a week later I was about to teach my morning class which Maze always attended but not today. After class Maze appeared to say hello to everyone and I went to the kitchen where she pushed me up against the same kitchen counter that I pushed her up against a week earlier and said I'm ready! That was a really exciting kiss and the day was filled with a sense of anticipation for what the night would bring. I think we were both really excited, we shared so much, we trusted each other so much but at the same time we were so relaxed about it. Maze suggested we wear the same dress, same colour, as we both shared a love of a certain brand of clothing and shared a love of many of the same styles which I would admit were geared probably for teenagers but were so cute I couldn't resist. Why would I let such a small detail bother me anyway, I've never really grown up when it comes to clothes or shoes. We both definitely had the same taste. Our hair coincidentally was about the same length and colour so when I took her by the hand and led her to my bedroom there was this amazing feeling of looking at myself 40 years ago.

We kissed and looked at each other in one of our intimate eye connecting exercises. We both agreed it was like looking into the past and the future simultaneously. One of the most spiritual and physically satisfying experiences I've had. She was incredibly beautiful in every way, shape and form. Rarely do we meet someone that we connect with on so many levels, a soul sister, a playmate, a lover, a daughter, a best friend. It felt so ephemeral, like two Goddesses who were playing together in the clouds. No boundaries, no self consciousness and no regrets. It was kind of perfect to use her words.

We both talked about the experience and we also talked about how much we enjoyed dating men so basically we were on the same page. What was this? We had no idea but we didn't need to know. We continued to date men and we continued caring about each other in an undefined way.

We had a pizza date one Saturday night with wine and dessert and both looked at each other on the drive home and said, my stomach hurts no intimacy tonight, let's wait and we both burst out laughing. It really was like reading each others minds and stomachs at the same time.

Always looking for adventure and new experiences we tried mushrooms together one night. We went to watch the sunset on the beach and took the shrooms and as we lay back in the sand we started watching the clouds form into animal shapes and the roar of the ocean getting louder and wilder until it was pretty deafening and starting to get dark. We walked home having no idea what would develop as the night drew on. At one point we put on loud music and danced wildly, really wild like wild women style. Afterwards I think I recall us sitting crossed legged on the tapestry carpet in the middle of the kitchen floor laughing. The red glass tiles on the kitchen walls were shimmering like I had never seen them shimmer before, very beautiful indeed. Light danced around the room and the music was beautiful and swirling in a new age compilation way!

I think it was me that took Maze by the hand and led her upstairs but for some reason we were kind of out of sync. Maze had taken much more than me and was very slowed down, I having taken a quarter of what she had was definitely speeding. Our energies were colliding rather than matching. Interestingly enough I didn't pick up on it but she did. I couldn't see her fear, maybe I just didn't want to or maybe I was just in my own world. We did agree that our energies weren't the same nor were our desires. We went to our respective rooms and both slept it off.

I think what we learned from this experience was that we shouldn't try to nail anything down, nor define it nor talk it to death but rather accept it with compassion and love and know that our love goes deeper than any one experience or deeper than anything that could be explained or deconstructed.

In the weeks to come we randomly kissed in the hall passing each other or the kitchen or the living room but we never went back to that space of intimacy. We both decided our relationship could not be defined or deconstructed and reconstructed, it was not Eastern nor Western, Sacred or Mundane as Elif Shafak speaks so eloquently about in the "Forty rules of love."

We couldn't be closer or more connected but we both date men and we both understand and accept this is where we need and want to be right now.

This was the note she left on the kitchen counter to let me know she was ready to explore intimacies together.

I'm ready…
Dance…meditate..surrender..
Lets meet in the kitchen at 8pm

(wear your wine coloured dress like mine)

CHAPTER THREE

Letting go...

I'm developing a deeper feeling and meaning of letting go, expecting nothing, living on the edge of not wanting or desiring in relationships. I'm challenging my own paradigm consistently and uncomfortably. I'm turning it inside out and upside down and finding that like a child pulling apart lego pieces and putting them back together to form new shapes and new meanings I'm doing the same with my relationships and I'm surprising myself with my ability to adapt.

With one person in particular named Dane I realised I'm looking at this relationship more deeply and seeing that for it to be satisfying I need to let go on a much deeper level, a level of total surrendering. This mirrors a statement that Dane made one night while together he said, you are great but I think you could surrender just a little more you are almost there. I was stunned, how could he have possibly realised something about me that I didn't even realise about me. I thought how could I possibly surrender anymore, I'm already so out there. But you know what? He was right, I resisted the urge to say you gotta be kidding me, and said, ok let me explore this. Of course, all after my initial shock and dismay but also not totally understanding that where I was going would lead me to physical, physiological, psychological, mental, emotional and spiritual letting go and surrendering. Or at least it would in my head but upon reflection, not in my heart.

So the actions of letting go on a deeper level had for me to do with non-attachment. Could I not only not need anything, ask for anything beyond our times together but really not even seek attention through communication after we were together? No texting and saying that was a beautiful night, looking forward to our next time together. Is this the kind of non-attachment I've read about, talked about and even practiced in other areas of my life through the yoga and meditation? Everything comes with practice so if I practice completely letting go once we have said good-bye after our time together could I not even desire to text: Hey Good Morning, have a beautiful day! Or Wow, did you see tonights sunset? Or I thought about you today while driving down a beautiful country road.

My first try of surrendering to Dane with non attachment was interesting as I didn't recognise that I couldn't withdraw vulnerability because its vulnerability that makes it real and intimate without that it just feels like sex. But is it possible to be vulnerable and practice non attachment? I'm experimenting so I don't actually know. My second time with Dane I couldn't really see any difference from the first time but I recognised that when he left in the middle of the night I had no reaction I was happy to see him come but equally happy to see him go and happy for him to be doing what he needed to do. I actually to be honest never slept well when he stayed the night and some nights I even laid awake for most of the night. The third time we were together with my new way of thinking and being it all came together naturally. We had an amazing intimacy and I felt I could totally surrender, ask for nothing and be non attached. I didn't ask him if he was staying the night or not. It really didn't matter but he did stay the night and I slept like a baby, he left the next morning and I was totally satisfied that we had arrived at the perfect place and balance of non-attachment, vulnerability, surrender and non-wanting. The intimacy was perfect, the care and loving kindness was perfect. Ask for nothing and receive everything. No future projections, and no time spent wondering when I would see him again. My heart knows I will so that is enough for me, when it happens again is one of the those things that we don't really need to know. We may want to know but we don't really need to know. We don't need to know everything this is one of our human insecurities we all struggle with but it is also one that with practice can be overcome and certainly once it's overcome we can stay in the present moment.

As a very feminine woman I am very right brained.

I am creativity and a free spirit…

I am passion…

I am yearning sensuality…

I am the sound of roaring laughter…

I am taste…

I am the feeling of sand on bare feet…

I am movement and vivid colour and the urge to paint on empty canvas…

I am boundless imagination … art, poetry, I sense. I feel.

I am everything I ever wanted to be….

I so resonate with this heavily right brained women and I am so totally her, can this person practice non-attachment in relationships? I wish the above words were mine but they are not its something I found somewhere years ago written on the side of a wall with no credit to anyone. I wrote it down and I read it to myself frequently.

I truly believe we can continue to look inward and change old patterns that take us deeper into the "rabbit hole of mysteriousness", after all until about 30 years ago we thought the brain was a hard-wired machine. We now know it's anything but that. We deeply understand

27

the brains ability to reorganise itself by forming new neural pathways throughout life….and we do this in response to new situations or to changes in the environment or to new challenges. We understand that our brains are very malleable. With the discovery of neuroplasticity our brains ability to selectively transform itself in response to certain experiences has proven to be one of the biggest paradigm shifts that neuroscience has seen in the past 30 years.

I began to investigate this through my creative movement while teaching yoga. Instead of repeating the same patterns or sequences always in the same chronological order I began to transit the postures through transition sequences or flow sequences. So the transitions or flow patterns had as much importance as the posture itself or the "journey was equally as important as the destination". I looked at the way these sequences challenged the brain which from what I have read begins to shrink as we get older but if given new sets of challenges it continues to grow. I looked at how it affected students memory, balance and disposition.

I laid music down as a bed to rest the movement on so students could get out of their heads and into their hearts and the "flow of life." I realised students weren't so critical of getting it perfect so therefore weren't as goal oriented and were more in the present moment. They weren't looking into the "past" which is only interpretation and a distraction or projecting into the "future" which is illusion and also a distraction but were deeply in the present moment if only to momentarily stretch their brains to pick up the sequences if nothing else in the beginning! Exercising the body and the brain all the while "growing the brain."

"If we are wired to thrive in the presence of the unknown"-saying no to fear, then you and I were given the ability through our biology to access large fields of information or large patterns of movement's or sequences. Greg Braddon says, "we also have the capability to access biological plasticity and genetic plasticity we as humans are the only ones who can access this and change this." "In other words we have the ability to self regulate our own biology we can become our own empowered master."

Who Are We?

But the stories we.......

Tell ourselves......

About ourselves.......and Believe!

Change your story

Change your life

Our stories are coded into us as children. My mother coded in the following story. She said to me, "Don't let anything happen to you, don't get hurt".

But, if you do get hurt make it quick healing and an unspectacular event!

Why did she unknowingly code this into me? Because my sister, brother and father were always getting hurt and landing in hospitals. She simply didn't have the time and energy to deal with one more family member who was hurt and in need of her attention. So she coded, "don't get hurt".

I would of course have liked to think this was remarkable "feminine wisdom" at play but it was just possibly remarkable "feminine survival" at play.

It's funny how many stories of coding I'm beginning to remember and wondering how much they have shaped this behaviour and belief system that I am constructing for myself. One of the most powerful codings I can recall and honestly think of quite often is overhearing my mother say to some friends of hers how good I was. I was very young and once again my brother and sister were a lot of work and were always getting not only hurt but into a lot of trouble. Now that I reflect on it they were having a damn good time in life, acting out, living on the edge and risk taking. I envied their wildness.

While they were doing this I was the good girl, not having a whole lot of fun because when you have to be good you have to also limit yourself to fun and spontaneity. My mother said to a group of her friends and in my presence, she is so good I can just give her a piece of paper to play with and she will sit in the corner and play for hours. She's never a problem!

I developed a taste for pleasing other people so maybe this is the beginnings of becoming the YES girl, not at all for the right reasons but it got me into the habit of saying YES. It's taken me a long time to shed the label of "good girl", I began to feel the restrictions of always having to please people, I actually started wanting to be bad. I think I was teaching myself that I could say YES to myself for a change, I could honour myself and please myself and that saying YES just wasn't for all others and not myself but saying YES was for me too!

So here comes the "Celestine Prophecy," giving me permission to say YES and for all the right reasons. As I mentioned in chapter two YES took me all around the world working and meeting phenomenal peoples. YES, was so conditioned in me that it was natural but what was new was all the fantastic and wonderful adventures that YES was giving me. I was loving it and I am loving it!

At the same time I'm still able to say YES to others and help to serve them. It's just far more balanced now as I can say YES to me and YES to all others. I'm loving the way this is shaping a new paradigm and new belief system for myself. I'm loving life and embracing it with such balance and when it gets out of balance I can recalibrate through adjusting my way of thinking and adjusting and stimulating my chakras. This chakra practice has given me such strength and focus. Through locating them with touch, through chanting the special sounds and letting the vibrations spin the wheels of energy, through seeing the colours and understanding their individualised mantras and last but not least through doing the movements that send the energy soaring through my spine.

These are the sounds:

Lam chakra 1 base of spine

Vam chakra 2 reproductive area

Ram chakra 3 solar plexus

Yam chakra 4 heart

Ham chakra 5 throat

Sham chakra 6 forehead

Aum chakra 7 crown

Visualising the corresponding colours or wearing them is also powerful:

Red

Orange

Yellow

Green

Blue

Purple and violet to luminous white. And this is still just the tip of the iceberg.

CHAPTER FOUR

My favourite Blue Chair......

Maze just reminded me about my favourite blue chair, how much I love it and talk about it how painterly it is with huge blooms of coloured flowers that look like they were painted with broad heavy strokes. How I talk about the blue chair but never really sat in the blue chair. My little dog picked the blue chair as his favourite place of sitting. The sunlight streams through the window and hits his face just right when he sits in the blue chair.

Now I've begun to sit there, its cosy and comfortable and I fit perfectly in it, I'm surrounded by swathing blue colour but for the most part I can't admire it for its beautiful colours and painterly designs. But, I can feel it now in all its comfort...

The Blue chair has begun to mirror my garden or my garden is mirroring my blue chair or they are mirroring one another, I'm not sure which but it probably doesn't matter. I've become a little obsessed with my garden. Planting beautiful colour in surprising places and creating a secret garden. The colours of violet pansies represent for me the crown chakra, the deep purple salvia are the 6th chakra and third eye. The blue throat chakra is seen in some tiny delicate blue flowers that hang perched at the end of long stalks and the green chakra well this heart chakra is everywhere in all shades of green from the most dynamic deep green to the lightest most delicate light green. Brilliant yellow appears in the wattle tree that hovers above the rose bushes it's so bright it almost hurts your eyes to gaze upon it, this is chakra 3. I have some wild flowers in bright orange these self seed and are popping their little heads up everywhere in the garden, they represent chakra 2. And last but not least the red chakra number 1 represented by big fat bright red blooms of the tomato Geranium.

My garden of chakras……my garden of intimacies…..my secret gardens …….my garden of gardens

I'm planting many things in my garden, choosing hopefully their most advantageous position for growth and happiness, I'm watering them, nurturing them and looking after them. When I pull them from their blue plastic pots I see many bound up roots crying to be untangled and given breathing space. As I put them in the prepared holes their roots almost start to breathe before my very eyes and then they spread and breathe a sigh of relief and then when I water them in they almost smile and give the thumbs up! I'm letting go and surrendering they say. I feel like I'm always letting go and surrendering and breathing sighs of relief. It's like we are mirroring one another. It's like one thing planted and one thing in my life goes. Is this a meaningful coincidence or a spiritual design. Some friends, family and acquaintances are leaving or dying. Both are deaths just different kinds of deaths. Again, another opportunity to deepen my belief system in "giving everything and asking for nothing", unconditional love and compassion, integrity and dignity, all currencies that matter and most of all recognising the depth of impermanence.

So, wow here I go lining up my work, my relationships, my creativity, with my deepening belief system. At the same time I'm challenging myself in deeper and more meaningful ways and in ways I never realised

I would have to challenge myself. Going deeper down the "rabbit hole of mysteriousness", and deeper down the "rabbit hole of the unknown".

I just had an amazing thought, while my hands are gliding across the keyboard of my computer Maze said, you can type! I thought for a minute, oh yes, I can really type properly, I know where all the keys are, I can type without looking, I learned to type properly in high school.

When I was in high school we had guidance counsellors who brought us into their office at the beginning of year ten to map out our courses that would take us into the future equipped with all the skills we might need to get a good job.

The question they asked us was basically, "what do you want to do when you grow up", I was one of those fortunate kids that really, really knew what she wanted to do, I had known this as long as I could remember.

So, when Ms Cortez asked "what do you want to do when you grow up?" I proudly answered, I want to dance I want to be a dancer! She looked at me with serious eyes and said that's nice but what do you want to do as a job or a career? I said, I want to be a dancer. She asked can you make a living doing this? I replied I don't know I guess so. Maybe? She remarked so if this being a dancer doesn't work out what else might you choose to do? I thought for only a second as I had something else as back up. I didn't want to do this as much as being a dancer but it was a close second and I was pretty passionate about it. So, I said probably a little too loudly I want to be in the circus! I guess Ms. Cortez was running a little low on patience at this point or maybe running a little short on time as she probably had many other high school students waiting to talk about what they wanted to do for the rest of their lives. I started to get the feeling she was thinking please God don't send me more like this one. But she managed to force out, "do you have any circus skills?" This was said with a bit of a roll of the eyes that I picked up on and I

35

said no not yet. She then remarked if neither of these work out for you wouldn't it be nice to have some nice skills to fall back on you know like practical skills. The word nice was starting to be a trigger for me, remember I was the nice child who would sit for hours playing with a piece of paper so I said like what? Like typing she chimed in if you can type you can be a secretary or a receptionist of some sort or assistant. I kindly declined as I knew for sure that I wasn't ever going to be any of the above.

But as the interrogations continued and she got more desperate to find some courses that could streamline me into some possible kind of job at least till I got married, I began to weaken. She needed me to choose something quick smart that would line up with the schools curriculum and more importantly give her a sense of achievement and also give her the feeling that she did her job well enough that I would be supported going into the future. She really was trying to help me I can see that now and I could see that then I just couldn't see myself needing anything remotely as far from dance or circus as typing. Ms. Cortez had sandy blonde hair arranged in a teased bouffant manner with a swirl in the front, she was one of the younger staff and besides being a guidance counsellor she taught PE. She was always dressed immaculately, straight lined tight skirts with matching blazer jackets. If the skirt was dark blue the jacket was perfectly matching in colour and fabric. If her skirt was beige her jacket was also beige.

The day I was being interviewed she had on a seer sucker matching suit. I remember the lines were light, light green with an off white background, I stared at the lines so long that my eyes began to glaze over and looking at the seer sucker stripes made me sleepy so maybe because of this or maybe because I took mercy on her I yelled out, sign me up for the typing course! Maybe Ms. Cortez had a crystal ball or just somehow knew these skills would come in handy at some point, somewhere in my life time I don't really know but I know I have to thank Ms. Cortez wherever she is.

Indeed this skill is making my stories come out faster and easier. Oh and also Ms. Cortez not only did I become a professional dancer and teacher but I also joined the Circus for one year flying high on the trapeze. A sheer joy until it interfered with my future in dance and I had to make the decision to give it up and devote totally and fully to Ballet and Contemporary dance training. I even hold a Masters of Fine Arts Degree in Dance and Choreography. So to all of you guidance counsellors never squash a kids dream no matter how silly and impractical they sound. But do encourage them to learn to type as you never know when it might come in handy!

Dance gave me a real voice, the little girl who never said no, or got into trouble or got hurt or caused a problem and was content with playing with a piece of paper for hours suddenly had a voice and could express through movement. And boy did she speak loudly and express herself deeply and fully. She couldn't get enough of it. It didn't matter whether she was asked to express happy, sad, scared or angry or any subtle aspects of these emotions she could express it. Choreographers wanted to work with her because she was keen to please but also very keen to grow and evolve through movement. And extremely capable of realising a choreographers vision. I now realise I was doing an enormous amount of self healing from childhood.

I am still evolving through movement. I am constantly challenging the parameters of how dance meets yoga and how yoga meets dance. I love testing the boundaries, deconstructing and reconstructing and trying to understand the relationships between all things living. Questioning and testing my limits and decoding life.

Movement for me has not only been my means of expression but my means of seeing the world and interpreting the world. We still have the deepest of relationships. I would have to say that without this means of expression I would not have found my voice on this page I truly don't believe I would have been able to flow across this page so easily. And very possibly I would not have had the courage or the creativity to create a new model and belief system for myself. I would possibly have not been able to facilitate and navigate multiple relationships with love and compassion, integrity and dignity. So, daily I bow down to dance and yoga to movement and expression and I give thanks.

CHAPTER FIVE

Expect the Unexpected......

So, I have an unexpected date in the midst of my other dating rituals. Not only was it unexpected but it was quite by accident. His name is Kai, I didn't realise he wasn't from my city of even State or I most likely wouldn't have gotten involved. So, as fate would have it we both swiped right and we were thrown together. By the time we could meet up he was back in his thriving city and I was back to my busy life in my little town. He wrote with a casual attitude and I simply said if you are ever back in town for work let me know. About six weeks later he was and we went out for coffee, we laughed and enjoyed each others company and when we parted he said, I'll stay for an extra day or two if you will go out with me again. Kai drove to the little country brewery close to where I live. We had a fun dinner together laughing and chatting and then parted ways.

Some interesting and different things about Kai, he loves to talk, he didn't make any sexual advances and his language wasn't filled with sexual innuendo's. Also, Kai didn't even kiss me at the end of our dates hum. This made me realise something was very different about him. Could he really be trying to get to know me? Who I am, what I'm doing, where I'm going?

Until now every date and I mean every date had pounced on me at the finish of our time together. I had gotten so used to this that I figured this is the "new" dating ritual and this happens to everyone pretty much everywhere in the world and pretty much all the time.

My other thought was maybe he just wants to be friends or maybe he is asexual. It actually didn't matter they were fun nights out and I was getting to know another fabulous human being. I think it was the next day he wrote: would you fly to my city and let me show you around for a few days or 3 or 4 or 5? I had a feeling I should go, ask no questions just go and see what the Universe throws my way. The one thing I felt strongly was that I would be safe and there would be surprises coming my way. So, I trusted and I said yes, how about 3 days? He thanked me for trusting him and I said I think we are trusting each other. I said jokingly you aren't an axe murderer are you? He said you aren't a bunny boiler are you?

This set the tone for the most fun repartee which lasted 3 days and until the moment I stepped on the plane to come back home. I can't remember having a holiday this much fun, I can't remember being with someone I so connected with, I can't remember being with someone I've laughed with and, I can't remember being with someone who would let me fed them bites of croissant in the hotel cafe knowing everyone was picking up on our intimacies and he didn't even flinch. I can't remember an intimacy that felt this right and complete with me exposing me fearlessly and him exposing his relaxed and easy yet fearless nature.

A gentleman that opens car doors, holds my hand while driving and calls me kitten. Who is this person I can't stop thinking about? That in itself is unusual, all other dates have had a beginning, middle and end with no projections to the future, all other dates have never truly allowed me to be me. I'm care free, free spirited and love an undramatic loving life style and relationship. Or maybe I have never completely felt safe being me. With Kai, I am me and I believe he is exactly who he is, no pretences. So, what is different is that there was a fuzzy beginning, a defined and beautiful present that we easily are able to navigate, an open ended future that neither one of us need to project to but we know in our hearts will be amazing when we do.

For the time we were together we wrapped our bodies around each other in bed and we fit perfectly, our intimacies were sweet, sexy and beautiful. For the first time in a long time I felt I could fearlessly taste the sweetness of orgasms with him, I could surrender totally and I could totally trust. I feel like I have met my soulmate! And you know me I didn't even believe there could possibly be such a thing as a single soulmate for each person. So, I'm watching my eleven year building of a belief system or a new paradigm crumble before my very eyes. But, the exciting thing is I have the opportunity to reconstruct a different and newer paradigm and I have no idea what it will look like, what colour it will be, what texture it will be and what shape it will take.

I'm free wheeling it, I'm deconstructing the old and reconstructing a newer more loving and fearless one. And i've never slept so well in my life.

Just before I'm ready to board the plane we look at our schedules and come up with some dates to see each other again. It wasn't but a few days after returning home that Kai rings and says how would you feel about me driving over next week! I want to see you. I issue an invitation somewhat casual saying sure, come ahead. Kai actually drives ten hours and arrives Thursday evening. It's almost winter and chilly so I make a fire and cook pasta with pesto. As we sit in front of the fire eating our pasta, drinking our wine and talking I realise I have never felt so comfortable with another human being. Who is this person I'm with that encourages me to be the fullness of who I am, The Warrior Women and the Goddess. Who is this person who makes reference to things that few people other than me would understand. Who is this

41

person who meets me on the level of music choices, old movies and even cartoons. He can be silly and laugh with me until we are almost crying. He meets my friends and connects with gentleness and ease as if he has known them forever. He makes love to me like I have never been made love to before with a sense of total surrendering in intimacy. No fearing, no game playing no holding back. He is emotionally mature, giving and fearless. He is certainly not an emotional procrastinator. He is anything but an emotional procrastinator. His heart is big and he makes decisions from his heart. He has a pureness and a childlike behaviour. He lives in the present moment and follows his heart with ease and comfort. At the end of our week together he looks at me and says, its only been a week and I've fallen deeply in love with you. My belief system crumbles even more. I'm on the verge of creating a new paradigm once again, one that is even more loving and risky and fearless and with the most extraordinary man.

Simultaneously, I get a call from my ex husband he has been given a diagnosis that is not looking so good. Bone cancer is the conclusion after many tests. A second opinion is sought after again, bone cancer. How long is any ones guess. To treat naturally or to submit to chemotherapy are his questions and his decisions to make right now. Does he look at quality of life and perhaps less time or look at perhaps extending his time with chemicals coursing through his body and sickness looming ahead. We have developed a lovely and loving friendship so we sit together each week and he tells stories. Some new stories that I've never heard before and perhaps wouldn't be hearing if he weren't dying and stories I've heard many times. Even some stories that shift his reality. I sit and listen as he carefully constructs with pain staking detail.

I wonder if he is using so much detail to test his memory and make sure he is not losing it.

Sometimes it's hard for him to remember a word and as he looks to the ceiling desperately searching for the word I wait, when I feel him get twisted by not being able to come up with the word I chime in and say you mean? And insert a word that I think he has been searching for, nine times out of ten I am able to find the word, he looks relieved, after all we lived together for thirty something years.

Some of his stories I was there for in real time but I hardly recognise them because he has shifted the reality so much that they are almost unrecognisable. And even though I was part of the story at the time I feel left out of the story now. And that's ok. Most of his stories are sad because they are about him being misunderstood by family, friends, lovers and work colleagues. Most of the stories he is not only misunderstood but also not appreciated.

Some of the stories are about him being victimised or even persecuted. He tells me about living life in the 60's when men were tough and expected to look and act a certain way. He talks about the fear and the feelings of always being on edge and not feeling free to express himself. I think this is what took him down the path of dance. There was a sense of freedom and safety in portraying something on stage that no one ever really knew whether it was you or a part you were playing. For him it felt more safe.

Marriage legitimised my ex husband and he loved that, two children further legitimised him and I know made him feel proud and worthy and enough and accepted. I played my role well but after awhile it had a high price, too high a price. I never felt comfortable in my role or like I could completely satisfy his needs. An undercurrent of sadness overtook the relationship that couldn't even be distracted by work or creativity anymore. I felt like I was suffocating in his sadness and control.

So, one morning I packed up my car and left and never returned. That was eleven years ago. It's taken years to find a loving friendship and balance but we have both worked on finding it and I believe have succeeded with sufficient honestly, integrity and authenticity.

I wake up early every morning. It would be the rare person that could beat me out of bed at 4:30am or the rare person that would even want to beat me out of bed at 4:30am in the morning! On the last morning of Kai's visit I wake up and realise I have never ever felt so comfortable and safe sleeping with anyone. I have never slept so soundly or deeply. I feel kind of shocked at this realisation and then I look over at him and I see Max my moodle sitting atop Kai's belly resting comfortably, relaxed and not only sound asleep but Max is snoring. Max is my barometer for authenticity and goodness. He tells me this is real, this person is here to stay so get comfortable and enjoy the ride. Max whispered to me, I like this man, I feel comfortable with this man.

It could be that this is the most fearless authentic ride I have taken for a very long time. I thought living the polyamorous life style of loving many was the most truthful and fearless thing I could do but now I actually think the unknown love that I'm embarking on now is the most truthful, outrageous and fearless thing I can do. It is the most beautiful thing I have witnessed so far, I'm blinded by its beauty. It's so shiny. So very, very shiny.

I feel so grateful for all the relationships that I've had over the past eleven years, they have made me "be here now." I'm grateful for these relationships bringing me to the place that I am at in this moment in time. I'm grateful for the people that have allowed me into their lives and who have allowed me to love them. I have learned to roll over, sit up, crawl and eventually walk through new ways of thinking and believing. I created a new paradigm for myself to live by and did so in the frame work of my own creativity and comfort. I thought I was creating, loving and living in the fullness of my "divine feminine "and my "warrior goddess" but now I KNOW I am. You know how I know?

I know because I have never been more sure of "Who I am," "Where I'm going" and "What I'm doing" and I have never felt more beautiful and comfortable in my own skin.

As Elif Shafak writes, "solitude is good for us as it means being alone without feeling lonely." "But eventually it is best to find a person, the person who will be your mirror. Remember only in another person's heart can you truly see yourself and the presence of God within you."